I0483804

The goal of the National Diabetes Education Program (NDEP) is to reduce the morbidity and mortality caused by diabetes and its complications through educational efforts that increase awareness of the seriousness of the disease and the value of its management and prevention. *Guiding Principles for Diabetes Care: For Health Care Professionals* is a key resource to help all health care professionals assure that they are providing current, quality diabetes care.

NDEP EXECUTIVE COMMITTEE

Francine Kaufman, M.D., Chair
Ann Albright, Ph.D., R.D.
Jeffrey Caballero, M.P.H.
Judith E. Fradkin, M.D.
Martha M. Funnell, M.S., R.N., C.D.E., Chair Elect
Lawrence Blonde, M.D., F.A.C.P., F.A.C.E., Immediate Past Chair

NDEP STEERING COMMITTEE MEMBERS

American Academy of Family Physicians
American Academy of Nurse Practitioners
American Academy of Pediatrics
American Academy of Physician Assistants
American Association of Clinical Endocrinologists
American Association of Diabetes Educators
American College of Physicians
American Diabetes Association
American Dietetic Association
American Medical Association
American Pharmacists Association
Association of American Indian Physicians
Association of Asian Pacific Community Health Organizations
Black Women's Health Imperative
Diabetes Research and Training Centers
Juvenile Diabetes Research Foundation International
Khmer Health Advocates, Inc.
Lions Clubs International
National Alliance for Hispanic Health
National Association of School Nurses

National Hispanic Medical Association
National Latina Health Network
National Medical Association
Papa Ola Lokahi
The Endocrine Society

FEDERAL LIAISONS TO THE NDEP STEERING COMMITTEE

Agency for Healthcare Research and Quality
Centers for Disease Control and Prevention/Division of Diabetes Translation
Centers for Medicare and Medicaid Services
Indian Health Service
Council of State Diabetes Prevention and Control Programs
Bureau of Primary Health Care, Health Resources and Services Administration
National Institutes of Health/National Institute of Diabetes and Digestive and Kidney Diseases
National Kidney Disease Education Program
U.S. Veterans Administration Health Care System

NDEP STAFF

Joanne Gallivan, M.S., R.D., Director, NDEP, NIH
Rachel Weinstein, M.Ed., Deputy Director, NDEP, NIH
Susan McCarthy, M.P.H., C.H.E.S., Acting Director, NDEP, CDC
Betsy Rodríguez, M.S.N., C.D.E., Acting Deputy Director, NDEP, CDC
Elizabeth Warren-Boulton, R.N., M.S.N., Liaison, Hager Sharp, Inc.

Technical reviewers for the content of this resource

W. Lee Ball, Jr., O.D., F.A.A.O.
Barbara Bartman, M.D.
Charles M. Clark Jr., M.D., NDEP Chair Emeritus
Judith Dempster, D.N.Sc., F.N.P., F.A.A.N.P.
Javier LaFontaine, D.P.M., M.Sc.
Margaret Gadon, M.D., M.P.H.
James R. Gavin III, M.D., Ph.D.
Amparo González, R.N., B.S.N., C.D.E.
J. Michael González-Campoy, M.D., Ph.D., F.A.C.E.
Mary Jo Goolsby, Ed.D., M.S.N., N.P-C, F.A.A.N.P.
JoAnn Gurenlian, R.D.H., Ph.D.

Sabrina Harper, M.S.
Joe Humphry, M.D.
Jane Kelly, M.D.
Sue Kirkman, M.D.
David Marrero, Ph.D.
Bob McNellis, M.P.H., P.A-C.
Andrew Narva, M.D.
Sandra Parker, R.D., C.D.E.
Christy Parkin, M.S.N., R.N., C.D.E.
Kevin Peterson, M.D.
Susan A. Primo, O.D., M.P.H., F.A.A.O.
Tanya Pagán Raggio Ashley, M.D., M.P.H., F.A.A.P.

Michael Parchman, M.D., M.P.H., F.A.A.F.P.
Leonard Pogach, M.D., M.B.A.
Donna Rice, M.B.A., B.S.N., R.N., C.D.E.
Julio Rosenstock, M.D.
Peter Savage, M.D.
Pamella Thomas, M.D., M.P.H., F.A.C.O.E.M., F.A.C.P.M.
Katherine R. Tuttle, M.D., F.A.S.N., F.A.C.P.
Sandeep Vijan, M.D., M.S.
Charlton Wilson, M.D.
Wilma Wooten, M.D., M.P.H.

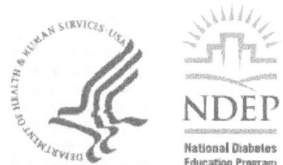

NDEP
National Diabetes
Education Program

The U.S. Department of Health and Human Services' National Diabetes Education Program is jointly sponsored by the National Institutes of Heath and the Centers for Disease Control and Prevention with the support of more than 200 partner organizations.

www.YourDiabetesInfo.org   1-888-693-NDEP (6337)   TTY: 1-866-569-1162

NIH Publication No. 09-4343   NDEP-16   Revised April 2009

Table of Contents

Introduction

These *Guiding Principles for Diabetes Care: For Health Care Professionals* provide an overview of the key elements of early and intensive clinical diabetes care and prevention. They form the basis of the National Diabetes Education Program's (NDEP's) public and professional awareness programs. The principles are based on the best level of evidence available, and key sources are noted. The NDEP adopts guidelines developed by the American Diabetes Association (ADA), and many have been incorporated into these guiding principles. Numerous other guidelines are available and some are noted in this document. It is essential that in practice, health care professionals focus on the similarities rather than the differences in diabetes-related guidelines. This document also provides links to supporting resources and further information.

As the proportion of both minority populations and people aged 60 and older increases in the United States, and the obesity epidemic continues, people with diabetes are becoming a larger part of the practices of family physicians and other primary care clinicians. Health care professionals involved in new or expanding diabetes care practices can use these guiding principles to ensure that they provide essential components of comprehensive diabetes care. In addition, health care payers, managed care organizations, and large employers can use this information to establish diabetes care principles and to assure quality diabetes care and treatment options in health plans.

NDEP encourages people with or at risk for diabetes and their families to participate actively with their health care team to plan and implement their care. While these principles serve as a guide for diabetes prevention and management, each person and his or her health care team should determine a specific prevention or management plan.

Team care is essential for effective diabetes prevention and management. Team structure is best determined by the practice setting. Teams should be led by the most appropriate health care professional, and may include primary care physicians, diabetes educators, endocrinologists, dietitians, nurses, nurse practitioners, pharmacists, physician assistants, psychologists, dental professionals, exercise professionals, social workers, specialists for care of the eye, foot, heart, and kidney, and others as necessary. Many of these team members also may be certified diabetes educators. Trained lay educators such as "promotores" and community health workers can be effective team members.

Other elements of importance to the delivery of diabetes care, in addition to team care, such as creating a patient registry, assessing practice needs, implementing processes of care, connecting to community resources, and evaluating outcomes are presented in detail on *www.BetterDiabetesCare.nih.gov*. This website provides tools and resources to help health care professionals implement systems changes.

Early identification and management of pre-diabetes can delay or prevent the onset of type 2 diabetes. In people with type 1 and type 2 diabetes, ongoing comprehensive diabetes care, including the ABCs of diabetes (A1C for glucose, Blood pressure, and Cholesterol), can prevent or control diabetes-related microvascular and macrovascular complications. With proper medical management, education, self-care, and attention to behavior, social, and environmental factors, people with diabetes and pre-diabetes can live long, active, and productive lives.

Identify People with Undiagnosed Diabetes and Pre-diabetes

To improve health outcomes it is essential to identify people at high-risk for diabetes, as well as those who are undiagnosed, and treat them appropriately.

Pre-diabetes occurs when a person's blood glucose level is higher than normal but not high enough for a diagnosis of diabetes (Table 1). People with pre-diabetes have impaired fasting glucose (IFG) or impaired glucose tolerance (IGT). Some people have both IFG and IGT. It is important to assess patients for pre-diabetes or diabetes so they can be treated effectively and monitored for disease progression. Identify people at high-risk based upon known risk factors (Table 2).

Consider testing plasma glucose if the person is:

- Age 45 or older
- An overweight adult with another risk factor (shown in Table 2).

Consider repeat testing at least every three years.[1]

TABLE 1. Definitions of Pre-diabetes and Diabetes [1]	
Pre-diabetes	
IFG	Fasting plasma glucose (FPG) 100–125 mg/dl after an overnight fast
IGT	2-hr post 75g glucose challenge 140–199 mg/dl
Diabetes	
	Random plasma glucose >200 mg/dl with symptoms (polyuria, polydypsia, and unexplained weight loss) **and/or**
	FPG>126 mg/dl* **and/or**
	2-hr plasma glucose>200 mg/dl* post 75g glucose challenge
	*Repeat to confirm on a subsequent day unless symptoms are present.

In 2007, at least 23.6 million Americans (7.8 percent of the population) had diabetes, of which 5.7 million had undiagnosed type 2 diabetes. At least 57 million U.S. adults have pre-diabetes, placing them at increased risk for cardiovascular disease and type 2 diabetes. [2]

Test plasma glucose in patients who have had hyperglycemia during acute illness or hospitalization, in people with cystic fibrosis, and in those on medications that predispose them to diabetes including anti-retroviral therapy for HIV, immunosupressants for transplantation, and atypical anti-psychotics. Inform these patients of their risk for diabetes and, if appropriate, encourage their actions to reduce risk as discussed in Principle 2.

Although the 2-hour 75g glucose challenge is more sensitive than a FPG value for diagnosing pre-diabetes or diabetes, use of the test is not always practical. If only a FPG is used, however, some diagnoses will be missed, particularly in elderly people. Clinical judgment should determine which test to use.

The diagnosis of pre-diabetes and diabetes should be clear, based on accepted guidelines for FPG or IGT values. **Avoid using terms with patients and their families, such as "a touch of diabetes" or "sugar is a little high" or "borderline diabetes" which suggest that diabetes is not serious.** People should know whether they have pre-diabetes, type 1 or type 2 diabetes, or if they have or had gestational diabetes. They also need to understand what the diagnosis means and the steps to take to lower their risk for progression to diabetes, or to manage their disease.

TABLE 2. Risk Factors for Type 2 Diabetes [1]

Overweight adult: Body Mass Index ≥25 kg/m2 (≥23 if Asian American or ≥26 if Pacific Islander) with one or more of the following:

- Family history: have a first-degree relative with diabetes
- Race/Ethnicity: African American, Hispanic/Latino, American Indian and Alaska Native, or Asian American and Pacific Islander
- History of gestational diabetes or gave birth to a baby weighing > 9 lbs
- Hypertension: blood pressure >140/90
- Abnormal lipid levels: HDL cholesterol level <35mg/dl; triglyceride level >250 mg/dl
- IGT or IFG: on previous testing
- Signs of insulin resistance: such as acanthosis nigricans or polycystic ovarian syndrome (PCOS)
- History of vascular disease: diagnosed by physical exam and testing
- Inactive lifestyle: being physically active less than three times a week

In the absence of the above risk factors, people age 45 and older are considered at risk and should be tested.

Note 1. The American Association of Clinical Endocrinologists (AACE) promotes risk factors that differ from the above as follows: hypertension >135/85; HDL cholesterol level < 40; history of *athero-sclerotic* vascular disease; women with PCOS – hyperadrogenism; and psychiatric illness. [4]

Note 2. The U.S. Preventive Services Task Force (USPSTF) concludes that the evidence is insufficient to recommend for or against routinely screening asymptomatic adults for type 2 diabetes, impaired glucose tolerance, or impaired fasting glucose. [5] The USPSTF recommends screening for type 2 diabetes only in adults with dyslipidemia or sustained blood pressure (treated or untreated) over 135/80, in whom knowledge of diabetes status would lead to different blood pressure goals, or those with intermediate scores on cardiovascular disease (CVD) risk engines in whom knowledge of diabetes status would trigger statin use. www.ahrq.gov/clinic/3rduspstf/diabscr/diabetrr.htm

Women with a history of gestational diabetes are at increased lifelong risk for diabetes. They should be tested for diabetes or pre-diabetes periodically as noted in Table 3:

TABLE 3. Case Finding Recommendations for Women with History of Gestational Diabetes [6]

TIME	TEST
Post-delivery (1–3 days)	Fasting or random plasma glucose (PG)
6 to 12 weeks postpartum	2-hr PG post 75g glucose challenge
1 year postpartum	2-hr PG post 75g glucose challenge
Annually	Fasting PG
Every three years and before another pregnancy	2-hr PG post 75g glucose challenge

For NDEP patient resources for diabetes prevention see page 22.

Manage Pre-Diabetes to Prevent or Delay the Onset of Type 2 Diabetes and Its Complications

People with pre-diabetes are at risk of developing type 2 diabetes and cardiovascular disease. As found in the Diabetes Prevention Program (DPP)[7], lifestyle interventions in people at high-risk can reduce their risk of developing type 2 diabetes by more than half. This powerful reduction in risk of type 2 diabetes affects all subgroups including men and women, high-risk racial groups, women with a history of gestational diabetes, and is even greater in people age 60 and older.

Progression to type 2 diabetes among people with pre-diabetes is not inevitable.

Disease progression

Progression to type 2 diabetes among people with pre-diabetes is not inevitable. About 5 percent of the lifestyle intervention group developed diabetes each year during the study period compared with 11 percent per year in those who did not get the intervention. People at risk for diabetes need to understand what pre-diabetes means and the steps to take to lower their risk for diabetes.

Children whose BMI is >85th percentile for their age are at increased risk for developing type 2 diabetes. They should be counseled to increase physical activity and reduce their rate of weight gain while allowing for normal growth and development.

High-risk older adults can significantly reduce their risk of developing **type 2** diabetes through lifestyle changes. The DPP found lifestyle interventions in people at high-risk age 60 and older reduced their risk of developing **type 2** diabetes by 71 percent. Medicare Part B now offers older adults preventive care benefits including a "Welcome to Medicare" physical exam, and diabetes and cardiovascular screening tests for people at risk. *www.cms. hhs.gov/MLNProducts/downloads/expanded_benefits_06-08-05.pdf*

Women with a history of gestational diabetes need to be counseled about their increased lifelong risk for diabetes and ways to lower their risk. **Children of women with gestational diabetes also are at increased lifelong risk for diabetes**. [8] The mother's history of gestational diabetes should be noted in the child's medical record. Breastfeeding may help prevent obesity in these children and may lower their risk for type 2 diabetes. Since fami-

lies share lifestyle habits, following a healthy lifestyle can benefit the mother and her children by lowering their risk for type 2 diabetes.

Lifestyle modification

Based on the DPP findings, NDEP promotes actions to prevent or delay the onset of **type 2** diabetes in people at risk and provides a toolkit for health care professionals. Lifestyle modification with a low-fat, reduced-calorie meal plan and increased physical activity should be discussed with all people who have pre-diabetes (Table 4). Refer to community resources whenever possible. (See Resource section for *Small Steps. Big Rewards. Your GAME PLAN to Prevent Type 2 Diabetes: Health Care Provider Toolkit* and *The Road to Health Toolkit* — a multi-component primary prevention resource.)

Medication therapy

To prevent or delay the onset of type 2 diabetes, therapy may include the insulin-sensitizing medication metformin for some people with pre-diabetes (Table 5). In the DPP, individuals with IGT who took metformin reduced their risk of developing diabetes by almost one-third. Metformin was more effective in younger, heavier people and less effective in people over the age of 60. [9] Metformin is not FDA approved for treatment of pre-diabetes.

Antihypertension and lipid-modifying medications and aspirin should be used to treat and modify cardiovascular risk as appropriate.

TABLE 4. Lifestyle Modification for Diabetes Prevention or Delay of Onset

Collaborating with patients to set short-term, specific, realistic goals can help support lifestyle change efforts.

Nutrition therapy:
- An integral part of a healthy, sustained weight loss program is the subtraction of calories each day from the diet. For most people, weight loss diets should supply at least 1,000 to 1,200 kcal/day for women and 1,200 to 1,600 kcal/day for men.
- Total fat should be 25 to 35 percent of total calories and saturated fat less than 7 percent.
- Portion control is essential for weight loss.

Physical activity:
- Patients should get at least 30 minutes of moderate-intensity physical activity five days a week. Daily activity time can be broken into segments. Brisk walking is an excellent form of moderate-intensity physical activity. *www.health.gov/paguidelines/default.aspx*
- NDEP provides tools to help people track their daily food, calorie, and fat intake, as well as physical activity.

Behavior therapy: [3]
- Knowledge is essential but rarely adequate to sustain behavior change over the long-term.
- Effective behavioral strategies that patients can use in their efforts to modify their lifestyles include: self-monitoring, stress management, stimulus control, problem-solving, self-directed goal-setting, cognitive restructuring, and social support.
- Behavioral therapies may help adoption of diet and activity changes.

Weight loss:
- Realistic yet clinically meaningful weight loss goals call for a 5 to 7 percent reduction in initial weight (10 to14 pounds (4.5 to 6.3 kg) for a 200-pound (90.6 kg) person).

Follow-up and referral:
- A focus on improved glucose and cholesterol levels, blood pressure, and self-esteem can reinforce the importance of lifestyle changes that lead to modest weight loss.
- Follow-up and monitoring of a patient's progress is essential.
- Referral to registered dietitians and weight control or wellness clinics can help patients maintain lifestyle changes.

Obesity medications and surgery

Weight loss medications approved by the FDA may be used *as part of* a comprehensive weight loss program that *includes meal planning and moderate intensity physical activity and behavior therapy* for people with a BMI >30 or >27 with concomitant obesity-related risk factors or diseases. Continual assessment of obesity drug therapy for efficacy and safety is necessary. [3, 10]

Weight loss surgery is an option in carefully selected obese adults and older adolescents who have completed growth (BMI >35 with comorbid conditions such as diabetes; BMI>50 or >40 with comorbid condition in adolescents) when less invasive methods of weight loss have been unsuccessful and the patient is at high risk for obesity-associated morbidity or mortality. [11, 12]

TABLE 5. Addition of Metformin to Lifestyle Changes [9]

The use of metformin may be considered in *addition to lifestyle changes* to prevent or delay the onset of diabetes in individuals with IFG *and* IGT *and* one or more of the following:
- Age <60 years
- BMI >35 kg/m²
- Family history of diabetes in first-degree relatives
- Elevated triglycerides
- Reduced HDL cholesterol
- Hypertension
- A1C >6.0 percent

Metformin is not FDA approved for treatment of pre-diabetes.

For NDEP patient resources for diabetes prevention see page 22.

PRINCIPLE 3:

Provide Ongoing Self-Management Education for People with Diabetes

Effective patient self-management is essential for people to live well with diabetes. It enables them to make informed decisions and to assume responsibility for the day to day management of their disease. Diabetes self-management education (DSME), also called diabetes self-management training, gives people with diabetes the knowledge, skills, and tools they need to effectively manage their diabetes. Ongoing support for coping with the daily demands of living successfully with diabetes is critical.

Self-management training

Diabetes educators and other health care team members provide DSME to address the educational, clinical, behavioral, and emotional needs of the individual patient in a supportive environment. Using a patient-centered approach engages the patient in active collaboration with the diabetes team and enables the patient to create a workable self-management plan based on age, school, or work schedule, as well as daily activities, culture, religious practices, competing priorities, family demands, eating habits, physical abilities, and health problems. These experts are able to help the patient achieve the highest possible level of self-care and quality of life.

Patients with severe visual impairment can learn self-management skills such as self-glucose monitoring, foot exam, and insulin use with the assistance of talking glucose meters and insulin dosing devices and by learning non-visual techniques. Organizations such as the National Federation of the Blind (*www.nfb.org*) offer resources and education support.

Education and ongoing support process

The overall objectives of DSME are to support informed decision-making, self-care behaviors, problem-solving, healthy coping and active collaboration with the health care team and to improve clinical outcomes, health status, and quality of life. While there is no one "best" education approach, programs that incorporate behavioral and psychosocial strategies demonstrate improved outcomes. Studies also show that culturally and age appropriate programs improve outcomes and that group education is effective. Standards for DSME have been developed through collaborative efforts of the key diabetes organizations. [13] In addition, the American Association of Diabetes Educators (AADE) identified seven self-care behaviors as a method for categorizing patient behaviors. (Table 6)

DSME is effective for improving metabolic and psychosocial outcomes, at least in the short term. As a result of DSME, people learn about diabetes and its management, define personal goals and strategies to reach those goals, make informed choices about therapies, develop behavioral and coping skills to support those choices, and evaluate the effectiveness of their efforts. Ongoing diabetes self-management support is critical for patients to sustain the gains made during DSME. [14]

Communication strategies

Effective communication can improve self-efficacy, support patients' behavior change efforts, and facilitate healthy coping. Effective strategies such as motivational interviewing are designed to assist patients to identify their own concerns, supports, and challenges and strategies to overcome barriers. Conversation maps are self-discovery learning tools that can help engage patients around self-management issues. For resources to help health care professionals enhance their communication skills, visit *www.betterdiabetescare.nih.gov/WHATpatientcenterededucation.htm; www.diabetesincontrol.com/issues/ issue317/about_healthyi.pdf.*

Financial Resources

Medicare covers diabetes self-management education from a recognized program, medical nutrition therapy from a registered dietitian, and diabetes equipment and supplies (i.e., blood glucose meters, test strips, and lancets). Other diabetes-related items covered include A1C and cholesterol tests, a dilated eye exam, glaucoma screening, flu and pneumococcal pneumonia shots, and a foot exam by a podiatrist if nerve damage is present. Medicare Part D offers prescription drug plans for enrollees. Most other insurance providers offer similar coverage for people with diabetes.

Recognition of quality care

To promote quality education for people with diabetes, the ADA recognizes programs that meet National Standards for Diabetes Self-Management Education Programs. The National Standards for DSME define quality diabetes self-management education and assist diabetes educators in a variety of settings to provide effective education. ADA and the National Committee for Quality Assurance also recognize physicians that voluntarily meet performance measures of adult or pediatric care. *www.diabetes.org/ for-health-professionals-and-scientists/recognition.jsp*

For NDEP resources for people with diabetes see page 22.

TABLE 6. AADE7 Self-Care Behaviors™: Summary of Diabetes Educator Assistance with Patient Self-Care Behaviors

Healthy eating

Diabetes educators help people learn about the effect of food on blood glucose and sources of carbohydrates, protein, and fat, make healthy food choices, adjust portion sizes, read labels, count carbohydrates, and plan and prepare meals.

Being active

Diabetes educators and their patients collaborate to address barriers, such as physical, environmental, psychological, and time limitations. They develop an appropriate activity plan that balances food and medication with the activity level.

Monitoring

Diabetes educators can instruct patients about self-monitoring blood glucose equipment choice and selection, timing and frequency of testing, target values, and interpretation and use of results. Patients are taught to regularly check their blood pressure, urine ketones, and weight, as appropriate.

Taking medication

The goal is for the patient to learn about each medication, including its action, side effects, efficacy, toxicity, prescribed dosage, appropriate timing and frequency of administration, effect of missed and delayed doses, and instructions for injection, storage, travel, and safety.

Problem solving

Collaboratively, diabetes educators and patients address barriers, such as physical, emotional, cognitive, and financial obstacles, and develop coping strategies.

Reducing risks

Diabetes educators assist patients in gaining knowledge about standards of care, therapeutic goals, and preventive care services to decrease risks. Skills taught include smoking cessation, foot inspections, blood pressure monitoring, self-monitoring of blood glucose, aspirin use, and maintenance of personal care records.

Healthy coping

Diabetes educators can identify the patient's motivation to change behavior, then help the patient set achievable behavioral goals, address barriers, and develop coping skills. The educator can assess patients for depression and refer for therapy.

www.diabeteseducator.org/ProfessionalResources/ AADE7

Provide Comprehensive Patient-Centered Care to Prevent or Delay the Onset of Diabetes Complications and to Treat Diabetes and Existing Complications

Good management of blood glucose (A1C*) levels can reduce symptoms related to diabetes and reduce the risk of both acute and chronic complications. Additional interventions to control blood pressure and cholesterol levels, along with smoking cessation, can significantly lower risk for long-term diabetes complications. The health care team should work in partnership with the patient to determine an individualized diabetes management plan, discussing options, goals, and individualized targets linked to the plan. Factors such as life expectancy, risk of hypoglycemia and the presence of advanced diabetes complications, or other medical conditions need to be taken into account when deciding which target values are most appropriate for an individual.

* NDEP and it partners have adopted the simple name "A1C" for the hemoglobin A1C test.

A major limitation to available data is that the optimum levels of control for particular patients are not identified, as there are individual differences in the risks of hypoglycemia, weight gain, and other adverse effects. Further, with multifactorial interventions, it is unclear how different components (e.g., educational interventions, glycemic targets, food selection, lifestyle changes, and medications) contribute to the reduction of complications. The level of evidence for a given guideline should be considered when individualizing targets.

Intensification of treatment over time is essential for people with type 2 diabetes so that they continue to meet therapeutic goals. It should be made clear that *progress* toward treatment targets is important since the absolute benefits lessen the closer one gets to the goal. Clinicians may choose to use health risk calculators such as Diabetes PHD (*www.diabetes.org/diabetesphd/default.jsp*) or the UKPDS Risk Engine (*www.dtu.ox.ac.uk/index.php?maindoc=/riskengine/*) to review estimates of the magnitude of absolute risk reduction as part of a treatment plan, especially in the context of intensifying treatment at values marginally above treatment goals. Treatment goals for A1C, blood pressure, and LDL-cholesterol that are recommended by the ADA and promoted by the NDEP are listed in Table 7.

Evidence for benefits of good blood glucose control

The Diabetes Control and Complications Trial (DCCT) [15] found that individuals with type 1 diabetes who achieved tight glucose control reduced microvascular complications up to 75% during the trial. The Epidemiology of Diabetes Interventions and Complications [16] follow-up study of participants in the DCCT showed that participants also had lasting benefits years later. Benefits included major reductions in eye, nerve, kidney, and heart complications with less than half the number of cardiovascular disease (CVD) events than the conventionally treated group.

Similarly, the 10-year follow-up of the United Kingdom Prospective Diabetes Study (UKPDS) [17] in people with type 2 diabetes found that although differences in glycemic control between intensive (A1C goal 7%) and standard treatment were lost within a year of the end of the original trial, significant microvascular benefits persisted at 10 years, and significant macrovascular benefits, including reduced myocardial infarction, emerged in the insulin/sulfonylurea group and persisted in the metformin group.

Findings from three other recent clinical trials (ACCORD, ADVANCE, VADT*) indicate that caution is needed in setting A1C goals lower than 7% in people with longstanding type 2 diabetes who have CVD or multiple CVD risk factors.

- In the ACCORD trial, over an average period of 3.5 years, more intensive blood glucose control ("near-normal" A1C goal < 6.0%) in older patients (mean age 62 years) with a 10 year average duration of diabetes and known CVD or with multiple CVD risk factors was associated with an approximately 20% increase in overall and cardiovascular mortality compared to standard glucose control (A1C goal 7.0-7.9%).
  - All three trials showed trends toward lower rates of non-mortality CVD outcomes with more intensive blood glucose control, but none were statistically significant.
- All three trials showed that more intensive glucose control increased the risk of severe hypoglycemia.
- Confirming earlier evidence, the ADVANCE trial showed that more intensive blood glucose control lowered the risk of new or worsening microvascular complications, particularly new onset microalbuminurea and new or worsening nephropathy.

* **ACCORD** – Action to Control Cardiovascular Risk in Diabetes [18]
ADVANCE – Action in Diabetes and Vascular disease: PreterAx and DiamicroN MR Controlled Evaluation [19]
VADT – Veterans Affairs Diabetes Trial [20]

Guiding Principles Based on the Above Findings and DCCT/EDIC and UKPDS

- Customary levels of intensive glucose control (A1C goal <7%) in newly diagnosed people with either type 1 or type 2 diabetes not only has benefits during the period of intensive therapy but also has a "legacy effect" in which microvascular and macrovascular benefits are maintained or realized years later.
  - Starting optimal blood glucose management as early as possible and maintaining it as long as possible with out inducing significant hypoglycemia in people with either type 1 or type 2 diabetes is beneficial.

- While the usual A1C goal for most people with diabetes is <7%, treatment must be individualized.
  - Less intensive control may be appropriate in older people; those with epilepsy; people with long-standing diabetes and CVD or multiple risk factors; those with advanced diabetes complications such as chronic kidney disease or autonomic neuropathy; or others at risk of severe hypoglycemia.
  - More intensive control to near-normal A1C levels may be appropriate for people with new-onset diabetes who have a long life expectancy and do not have CVD or multiple risk factors, or other co-morbidities, that increase risk of hypoglycemia or other adverse effects of treatment.

Evidence for blood pressure control

Blood pressure reduction also substantially improves clinical outcomes. In the UKPDS, tight blood pressure control which targeted <150/85 (achieved 144/82 mmHg) compared to a target of 180/105 significantly reduced risk for diabetes-related deaths, stroke, heart failure, microvascular disease, retinopathy progression, and deterioration of vision in people with type 2 diabetes. [21] However, in the 10-year follow up of the UKPDS [22], differences in blood pressure control were lost within two years of the end of the original trial, and at 10 years there was no difference in outcomes attributable to blood pressure control. **These finding indicate that benefits of blood pressure control do not extend beyond the period of intensified therapy, and ongoing treatment is essential.**

The effectiveness of reducing diastolic treatment goals in people with diabetes was demonstrated by the Hypertension Optimal Treatment study that found a 51 percent reduction in major cardiovascular events at a diastolic goal of 80 mmHg compared with 90 mmHg. [23] These findings together with epidemiologic evidence led to the ADA recommended blood pressure level of 130/80 for people with diabetes. The ongoing ACCORD trial will provide additional information on whether a systolic BP target <120 has better outcomes than a target <140 mmHg in patients with type 2 diabetes.

The Systolic Hypertension in Elderly Program study found that diuretics reduced cardiovascular death in people with diabetes by 31 percent. [24] Angiotensin converting enzyme (ACE) inhibitors have been demonstrated to provide substantial benefits, including reduced risk of heart attack, stroke, or cardiovascular death [25, 26] and prevention of progression of nephropathy. [27] The recent ADVANCE study assessed the effects of the routine administration of an ACE inhibitor-diuretic combination in patients with diabetes and found a significant reduction in relative risk of a major macrovascular or microvascular event, death from cardiovascular disease, and death from any cause. [28]

Evidence for lipid control

People with diabetes commonly have lipid patterns characterized by elevated triglyceride and reduced HDL-cholesterol levels. While their LDL-cholesterol values are generally not higher than those in non-diabetic individuals, there is often a greater proportion of smaller, denser and more atherogenic LDL particles. [29] Studies using the HMG-CoA reductase inhibitors (statins) have clearly shown that rigorous LDL-cholesterol reduction therapy can reduce the risk of CVD in people with diabetes.[30-33] Current guidelines recommend LDL-cholesterol less than 100 mg/dl in patients with diabetes. Some experts recommend optional, more aggressive lowering (<70 mg/dl) in patients with clinical CVD or at high risk of CVD. [1]

Multiple risk factor reduction

In the Steno-2 Study [34], a target-driven, long-term, intensified intervention aimed at multiple risk factors in patients with type 2 diabetes and microalbuminuria, the risk of cardiovascular and microvascular events was reduced by about 50 percent. This study clearly demonstrated the value of addressing A1C, BP, and LDL-cholesterol, the ABCs of diabetes. Long-term follow-up of the participants found significant sustained reductions in cardiovascular deaths. [35]

Weight loss

One-year data from the Look AHEAD (Action for Health in Diabetes) study [36] show that intensive lifestyle intervention in people with diabetes for weight loss through changes in diet and physical activity reduced body weight, A1C, systolic and diastolic blood pressure, and triglycerides, and increased HDL cholesterol. Fewer diabetes and anti-hypertensive medications were needed in the intensive intervention group. This ongoing trial will determine the effects of weight loss on long-term complications of type 2 diabetes.

Blood glucose management

As noted, the risk for microvascular and macrovascular complications of both type 1 and type 2 diabetes can be reduced by maintaining A1C close to 7%. The absence of symptoms of high blood glucose is an unreliable guide for judging glucose control, since symptoms do not occur until blood glucose reaches high levels. Diabetes is often called a "silent disease" because it can cause serious complications without having serious symptoms. The initiation and adjustment of therapy needs to target metabolic control as close to goal as possible without compromising patient safety. Patients on insulin or oral agents that stimulate insulin secretion are likely to have an increasing risk of hypoglycemia with an A1C below 7. Medical nutrition therapy and physical activity are essential from diagnosis onward for people with diabetes. For type 1 diabetes insulin is required at the onset of disease. For people with type 2 diabetes, the addition of metformin, combination therapy with other glucose-lowering medications, basal insulin, and prandial insulin, may become necessary over time to maintain the target A1C. Algorithms can help guide therapy selection. [39]

TABLE 7. ABC Treatment Goals for People with Diabetes [1] [37]

A1C <7.0 percent for patients with diabetes, in general*

Plasma blood glucose:

Preprandial capillary plasma glucose 70–130 mg/dl

Peak postprandial capillary plasma glucose <180 mg/dl (usually 1 to 2 hours after the start of a meal)

Be alert to the impact of hemoglobin variants on A1C values. For information see www2.niddk.nih.gov/variants

Blood Pressure <130/80 mmHg (if it can be achieved safely)

Cholesterol – Lipid Profile (mg/dl)
LDL <100 (for those with CVD <70)
HDL Men >40 Women >50
Triglycerides <150

***Individualize target levels** as appropriate. For example consider:
- A1C target as close to normal as possible without significant hypoglycemia in selected individuals such as those with short duration of diabetes, little comorbidity and long life expectancy.
- Less strict A1C target for people with severe hypoglycemia, limited life expectancy, comorbid conditions, advanced micro- or macrovascular complications, or long-standing diabetes.

Note 1. Similar recommendations for A1C, blood pressure, or cholesterol are available from:
- AACE (www.aace.com/pub/pdf/guidelines/DMGuidelines 2007.pdf)
- JNC7 the Seventh Report of the Joint National Committee on Prevention, Detection, Evaluation, and Treatment of High Blood Pressure (www.nhlbi.nih.gov/guidelines/hypertension/)
- National Kidney Foundation (www.kidney.org/professionals/KDOQI/guidelines.cfm) and the National Kidney Disease Education Program (www.nkdep.nih.gov/)
- National High Blood Pressure Education Program (NHBPEP) (www.nhlbi.nih.gov/about/nhbpep/)
- National Cholesterol Education Program (www.nhlbi.nih.gov/about/ncep/)
- American College of Physicians: Glycemic control and type 2 diabetes mellitus: the optimal hemoglobin A1c targets (www.annals.org/cgi/reprint/147/6/417.pdf); Lipid control in the management of type 2 diabetes mellitus (www.annals.org/cgi/reprint/140/8/644.pdf); The evidence base for tight blood pressure control in the management of type 2 diabetes mellitus (www.annals.org/cgi/reprint/138/7/587.pdf)

Note 2. A comprehensive assessment of North American and United Kingdom Glycemic Control Guidelines commissioned by the American College of Physicians is available. [38]

A1C values [40] and self-monitoring of blood glucose (SMBG) should be used to guide therapy to achieve glycemic targets. A1C is a standardized blood test that indicates the average blood glucose over the previous 8 to 12 weeks. People with diabetes should know their own A1C values (which may be interpreted by a calculated estimated average glucose or eAG) to determine whether they are reaching their targets. Labs may provide both A1C and the eAG equivalent. (See box below for conversion table and reference 40 for further information.)

Regular SMBG may help with self-management, such as changing medications, particularly for individuals taking insulin. SMBG can also be used to assess symptoms of hypoglycemia and hyperglycemia. Individual circumstances will define how often self-monitoring is used, the specific testing method, and the way to record and report results.

Both measures of long term control (A1C along with eAG) and measures of SMBG are valuable for assessing the adequacy of glycemic control and adjusting medications in patients with diabetes. While the A1C level gives an overall estimate of control over several weeks, the SMBG values can assess the variability of short term glucose levels. The latter may be important to reduce

post prandial hyperglycemic excursions or to confirm symptomatic or otherwise unrecognized hypoglycemia. During unstable periods, patients may need to increase the frequency of SMBG determinations.

For type 1 diabetes, basal and meal-related insulin doses may be prescribed several times a day via multiple injections or an insulin pump in an attempt to normalize glucose metabolism and simulate normal insulin physiology. Several types of glucose-lowering medications are available for the treatment of type 2 diabetes. These medications differ by their mechanism of actions that serve to: enhance endogenous insulin secretion, inhibit excessive hepatic glucose production, enhance insulin sensitivity in muscle and adipose tissue, delay gastrointestinal carbohydrate absorption, delay gastric emptying, inhibit glucagon secretion, and enhance satiety. These medications may be prescribed alone or in some combinations to meet treatment goals. Medications used to treat patients with diabetes are summarized on the NDEP website. (See Resource section for *Working Together to Manage Diabetes: Diabetes Medications Supplement*).

It has been shown that endogenous insulin levels decrease over time in people with type 2 diabetes, and most patients eventually require insulin replacement therapy if they are to attain and sustain glycemic targets. Informing these patients that beta cell function decreases over time, may help prepare them for the moment when the addition of insulin therapy may become necessary. It is critical that patients understand the importance of insulin therapy and the dangers of postponing its initiation when oral medications are no longer effective. The use of more predictable short and long-acting insulin analogs significantly reduces risk of hypoglycemia. Pen delivery devices also facilitate insulin administration and acceptance of insulin therapy.

Clinicians are encouraged to rely upon systematic reviews of the comparative effectiveness of glucose-lowering medications and insulin from sources such as the Agency for Healthcare Quality and Research [41] and Cochrane reviews (*www.cochrane.org/reviews:* Long-acting insulin analogues versus NPH insulin (human isophane insulin) for type 2 diabetes mellitus. Cochrane Database Syst Rev. 2007 Apr 18;(2):CD005613).

Note that in the hospital setting, effective glycemic control is important in order to improve patient outcomes. [1]

Results of the A1C-Derived Average Glucose study affirmed the existence of a linear relationship between A1C and average blood glucose levels. As a result, the ADA is promoting use of estimated average glucose or eAG. Patients will be able to receive A1C% and/or eAG values that relate to blood glucose values in mg/dl.

Formula 28.7 X A1C – 46.7 = eAG.

CONVERSION TABLE		
A1C	eAG	
%	mg/dl	mmol/l
6	126	7.0
6.5	140	7.8
7	154	8.6
7.5	169	9.4
8	183	10.1
8.5	197	10.9
9	212	11.8
9.5	226	12.6
10	240	13.4

Lipid and blood pressure management

Dyslipidemia and hypertension commonly coexist with type 2 diabetes and are clear risk factors for cardiovascular disease; and diabetes itself confers independent risk. Extensive trial evidence shows the efficacy of lipid-lowering therapy and targeted treatment of hypertension to prevent or slow cardiovascular disease onset in people with diabetes.

Lipid and blood pressure levels should be treated more aggressively in patients with diabetes than in the general population [1] because of the increased risk of cardiovascular and kidney diseases. Clinical trials have demonstrated clear benefits of hypertension control on both macro- and microvascular complications of diabetes. In addition, significant benefits of lowering LDL-cholesterol have also been demonstrated in clinical trials conducted in patients with diabetes. Taken together, improved management of glucose, blood pressure and LDL-cholesterol, along with abstinence from smoking, can lead to major reductions in the risk of both small and large vessel complications associated with diabetes. [1]

Lipid management

To reduce the risk of cardiovascular disease, blood lipids need regular measurement and effective management — especially high LDL cholesterol, high total cholesterol, and low HDL cholesterol. Statins are the initial medications of choice for most people with elevated LDL cholesterol.

- Lifestyle modification to reduce saturated fat, *trans* fat, and cholesterol intake; weight loss (if indicated); and increased physical activity should be recommended.
- Statin therapy should be added to lifestyle therapy, regardless of baseline lipid levels, for diabetic patients with overt CVD and those without CVD who are over the age of 40 and have one or more other CVD risk factors.
- For lower-risk patients without overt CVD and under the age of 40, statin therapy should be considered in addition to lifestyle therapy if LDL cholesterol remains >100 mg/dl or in those patients with multiple CVD risk factors.
- In individuals without overt CVD, the primary goal is an LDL cholesterol <100 mg/dl.
- In individuals with overt CVD, a lower LDL cholesterol goal of <70 mg/dl, using a high dose statin, is an option.

Blood pressure management

Blood pressure management has been proven to reduce both microvascular and macrovascular diabetes complications. Control of hypertension is essential in order to reduce cardiovascular risk and kidney and eye disease risk.

- Strategies to reduce sodium intake and excess body weight, such as increasing consumption of fruits, vegetables, and low-fat dairy products, avoiding excessive alcohol consumption, and increasing activity levels, may have antihypertensive effects similar to pharmacologic monotherapy.
- In individuals with diabetes and mild hypertension (systolic blood pressure 130–139 mmHg or diastolic blood pressure 80–89 mmHg), an initial trial of nutrition and physical activity therapy may be reasonable.
- If the blood pressure is 140 mmHg systolic and/or 90 mmHg diastolic at the time of diagnosis, pharmacologic therapy should be initiated along with nutrition and physical activity therapy.

Medications used in the treatment of hypertension include thiazide diuretics, ACE inhibitors, angiotensin receptor blockers (ARBs), ACE inhibitor-diuretic combinations, beta blockers, and calcium channel blockers. Multidrug therapy usually is required to achieve and maintain a blood pressure goal of <130/80 mmHg that is recommended for most people with diabetes. At every visit to the health care team, blood pressure should be measured and treatment adjusted if necessary.

Other components of comprehensive diabetes care include (in alphabetical order):

Anti-platelet therapy [1]

Using aspirin therapy (75–162 mg/day) is recommended as a prevention strategy for cardiovascular events in those patients with diabetes who have a history of CVD or are at high CVD risk.

Dental care

Poor glycemic control may exacerbate periodontal disease and tooth decay. Conversely, periodontal disease may cause deterioration of glycemic control. All patients with diabetes should be encouraged to brush and floss their teeth after every meal, and to have professional dental cleaning at least once a year.

Depression management

The presence of diabetes may double the risk of depression. The risk increases as diabetes complications worsen. People who are depressed are less able to carry out self-management tasks. Screening for depression and treating it effectively can help improve diabetes management. The Patient Health Questionnaire (PHQ)-9 is a brief 9 item depression self-report scale that is an effective tool used to screen and diagnose depression as well as to monitor response to therapy. *http:// www.ihs.gov/MedicalPrograms/ Diabetes/resources/ bp06_DepressionCare.pdf*. Treatment of depression with psychotherapy, medication, or a combination of these treatments can improve a person's well-being and ability to manage diabetes. Treatment should be provided in accord with current mental health guidelines and in collaboration with the diabetes care team.

Kidney disease management [1]

Chronic kidney disease is defined as the persistent (at least 3 months), and usually progressive, reduction in estimated glomerular filtration rate (eGFR) to less than 60 mL/min/1.73 m^2, and/or albuminuria (a urinary albumin-to-creatinine ratio >30/mg/g). Kidney status should be annually assessed by a marker of damage, "spot" urine albumin-to-creatinine ratio, and an estimate of function, the eGFR, calculated from the serum creatinine level *http://nkdep.nih.gov/professionals/gfr_ calculators/ index.htm*.

Treatment with an ACE inhibitor or an ARB is recommended for patients with diabetes and hypertension and/ or albuminuria greater than 300 mg/day. These drugs may also be beneficial in normotensive patients with albuminuria between 30-300 mg/day, but data to support the routine use of ACE inhibitors in this setting does not yet exist.

Complications of kidney disease correlate with level of kidney function. When the estimated GFR is less than 60 ml/min per 1.73 m^2, screening for anemia, malnutrition, and metabolic bone disease is indicated. Early vaccination against hepatitis B is indicated in patients likely to progress to end-stage kidney disease.

Consider referral to a physician experienced in the care of kidney disease when there is uncertainty about the etiology of kidney disease (active urine sediment, absence of retinopathy, or rapid decline in GFR), difficult management issues, or advanced kidney disease. The threshold for referral may vary depending on the frequency with which a provider encounters patients with significant diabetic kidney disease. Consultation with a nephrologist when stage four chronic kidney disease develops has been found to reduce cost, improve quality of care, and keep people off dialysis longer.

Nonrenal specialists should educate their patients about the progressive nature of diabetic kidney disease; the renal preservation benefits of aggressive treatment of blood pressure, blood glucose, and hyperlipidemia; and the potential need for renal replacement therapy.

Medical nutrition therapy [42]

Medical nutrition therapy (MNT) is an integral component of diabetes management. MNT is usually provided by a registered dietitian who assesses a patient's nutritional status and collaborates with the patient to develop a personal meal plan. People with diabetes should be referred for MNT as needed to achieve weight and other treatment goals. For most people with diabetes, diet composition recommendations include total fat about 30 percent of total calories and saturated fat less than 7 percent. Intake of *trans* fat should be minimized. Monitoring carbohydrate intake is a key strategy in achieving glycemic control, whether by carbohydrate counting or experience-based estimation.

Weight loss is an important goal in overweight or obese individuals who have type 2 diabetes. Measuring waist circumference and the body mass index can help assess and monitor the level of adiposity. Heart disease risk increases with a waist measurement of over 40 inches in men and over 35 inches in women. Weight loss requires a reduction in energy intake and is enhanced by physical activity. A moderate decrease in caloric balance (500–1,000 kcal/day) will result in a slow but progressive weight loss (1–2 lb/week). For most people, weight loss meal plans should supply at least 1,000–1,200 kcal/day for women and 1,200–1,600 kcal/day for men.

Neuropathy management [1]

The early recognition and appropriate management of neuropathy is important because a number of treatment options exist for symptomatic diabetic neuropathy. Most common among the neuropathies are chronic sensorimotor distal symmetric polyneuropathy (DPN) and autonomic neuropathy. Up to 50 percent of DPN may be asymptomatic, and patients are at risk of insensate injury to their feet. Autonomic neuropathy may involve every system in the body and cardiovascular autonomic neuropathy causes substantial morbidity and mortality. Optimal glycemic control may slow progression, but not reverse, neuronal loss. Effective symptomatic treatments are available for some manifestations of DPN and autonomic neuropathy.

- All patients should be screened for distal symmetric polyneuropathy (DPN) at diagnosis and at least annually thereafter, using simple clinical tests.
- Educate all patients about self-care of the feet. For those with DPN, enhanced foot care education is necessary as well as referral for special footwear. Research indicates that patients at high risk of foot ulcers can be identified and taught self-management skills that can prevent ulcers and amputations. See Resource section for *Feet Can Last a Lifetime Kit* – a comprehensive kit for health care professionals that contains ready-to-use foot exam forms, Medicare certification forms for therapeutic footwear, a sample disposable sensory testing monofilament, and reproducible patient education materials.
- Screen for signs and symptoms of autonomic neuropathy at diagnosis of type 2 diabetes and 5 years after the diagnosis of type 1 diabetes.
- Medications for the relief of specific symptoms related to DPN and autonomic neuropathy are recommended, as they improve the quality of life of the patient.

Obesity treatment

Medication therapy for weight management may be considered part of the ongoing treatment for all patients with diabetes who are overweight or obese.

Bariatric surgery may be considered in obese (BMI >35) patients with diabetes who have not responded to medical management. The benefits and risks of bariatric surgery vary dependent upon individual circumstance, type of surgical procedure, and skill of the surgeon.

Physical activity

To improve glycemic control, assist with weight maintenance, and reduce cardiovascular disease risk, adults with diabetes, in consultation with their health care team, need:

- At least 150 min/week of moderate-intensity aerobic physical activity (50–70 percent of maximum heart rate)
and/or
- Seventy-five to 90 min/week of vigorous aerobic exercise (>70 percent of maximum heart rate)

Encourage patients to set a modest initial physical activity goal. Gradually increase the duration and frequency to 30 to 60 minutes of moderate aerobic activity, 3 to 5 days per week. Activity time can be spread out over each day.

Adults with diabetes, in the absence of contraindications, are advised to perform resistance exercise three times a week, targeting all major muscle groups, progressing to three sets of 8 to10 repetitions at a weight that cannot be lifted more than 8 to 10 times [43] and to follow guidelines shown at *www.health.gov/paguidelines/default.aspx*.

Children and adolescents need

- Sixty minutes or more of moderate or vigorous intensity aerobic physical activity every day
- On at least three days per week, muscle-strengthening (e.g., using playground equipment, climbing trees, and playing tug-of-war) and bone-strengthening activity (e.g., running, jumping rope, basketball, tennis, and hopscotch)

To sustain long-term weight loss, adults with diabetes need

- At least 60 minutes per day of moderate activity such as brisk walking, or 30 minutes per day of vigorous activity such as jogging, and
- To be assessed for risk of cardiovascular disease or injury, or contraindications for certain types of exercise, before beginning a vigorous physical activity program [44]

Retinopathy management

Optimal glycemic and blood pressure control can reduce risk of retinopathy or slow its progression. Patients should be monitored by an ophthalmologist or optometrist for retinopathy through annual dilated eye exams (if normal, the eye care specialist may advise an exam every two to three years). Most retinal eye disease can be treated successfully by laser therapy. Patients with any level of macular edema, severe background retinopathy, or any proliferative retinopathy should be referred for treatment to an ophthalmologist experienced in the care of retinal disease. Retinopathy is not a contraindication to low-dose aspirin use for CVD prevention.

Self-care behaviors

All people with diabetes need to work with their health care team to develop a personal food and physical activity plan and to attend to other self-care behaviors. Prevention of long-term complications is enhanced if people with diabetes practice the following healthy self-care behaviors:

- Eat a variety of foods high in fiber, low in sodium and sugar, and low in saturated and *trans* fats.
- Reduce food portion sizes to help with weight loss, if appropriate.
- Get 30 to 60 minutes of moderate–intensity physical activity most days of the week. This could be brisk walking, yard work, and actively playing with children, such as riding bicycles or playing soccer.
- Take prescribed medications, including low-dose aspirin, even when feeling good, with no symptoms.
- Check their blood glucose as advised and use the results to manage blood glucose.
- Check their feet daily and contact their doctor if a sore does not begin to heal after one day.
- Brush their teeth twice a day and floss once a day.
- Make regular visits to their health care team for diabetes, foot, dental, and eye care. Contact their health care team about any foot, dental, or eye problems.
- Seek help to stop smoking.
- Seek help for stress, diabetes-related distress, and depression.

Smoking cessation

Smoking more than doubles the risk for cardiovascular disease in people with diabetes. People who stop smoking greatly reduce their risk of premature death. Medications, counseling, and smoking cessation programs increase the chances of success, as do telephone help lines. Additional effective therapies include nicotine replacement products (e.g., gum, inhaler, and patch) *www.smokefree.gov*; 1-800-QUITNOW (1-800-784-8669) routes callers to their state's smoking cessation quit line or to the National Cancer Institute's quit line.

Vaccinations

- Provide influenza (annually).
- Provide pneumoccal (usually only once, repeat if over 64 or immunocompromised and the last vaccination was more than 5 years ago).

For NDEP resources for people with diabetes see page 22.

Consider the Needs of Special Populations — Children, Women of Childbearing Age, Older Adults, and High-Risk Racial and Ethnic Groups

Certain populations — children, women of childbearing age, the elderly, and different racial and ethnic groups — have special diabetes management issues that need to be addressed.

Diabetes in children

Diabetes is one of the most common chronic conditions in school-age children in the United States. About 183,300 youth under 20 years of age have diabetes – 0.2 percent of all in this age group. [2] Type 1 diabetes accounts for most cases. Type 2 becomes increasingly common after age 10, with higher rates in minority groups than in non-Hispanic whites. The highest rates are seen in American Indian youth. As more children and teens become over-weight, a hybrid form of diabetes may become more common. Youth with hybrid diabetes are likely to have both insulin resistance that is associated with obesity and type 2 diabetes, and antibodies against the pancreatic islet cells that are associated with autoimmunity and type 1 diabetes. In addition to lifestyle changes, treatment may involve both insulin therapy and oral glucose-lowering medications.

The treatment of children with diabetes differs from that of adults since attention must be paid to physical growth and maturation, decreased insulin sensitivity during mid to late puberty, ability to provide self-care, the need to provide care at school, neurological vulnerability to hypo-glycemia in young children, and the eventual need to transition to adult care. Cardiovascular disease risk factors have been observed among some youth with both type 1 and type 2 diabetes. Evidence indicates that primary prevention of cardiovascular disease should begin in childhood. [45]

Management and education

Education of the family about their child's diabetes management is essential. The family and their diabetes care team need to develop individualized blood glucose targets, types and doses of insulin, frequency of blood glucose testing, when to test for ketones, insulin delivery systems, and details of dietary management. Other essential management tasks include recognition of high and low blood glucose, confirmation by blood glucose testing when possible, and, where necessary, prompt administration of glucose to treat hypoglycemia (or glucagon for severe hypoglycemia).

Most young people can learn to adjust their insulin doses according to activity and eating patterns — rather than follow a rigid meal plan and insulin dose schedule. Insulin may be injected three or more times a day or may be given by an insulin pump that provides continuous subcu-taneous infusion of basal and meal-related doses of insulin. Children may learn to vary their carbohydrate intake and calculate the proper insulin dose by using an insulin/carbohydrate ratio.

Diabetes at school

The health care team needs to work with the school nurse to provide a written diabetes management plan for every student with diabetes. The plan must be conveyed to the school nurse or trained school personnel who will work with students and parents to implement the plan in the school setting. Children with diabetes should be able to participate fully in all sports and physical education activi-ties and to attend field trips. (See Resource section for *Helping the Student with Diabetes Succeed: A Guide for School Personnel*.)

Psychosocial issues

Learning to cope with the disease often causes emotional and behavioral challenges, sometimes lead-ing to depression or eating disorders. A social worker or psychologist may help young people and their families learn to adjust to the lifestyle changes needed for effec-tive diabetes management. As teenagers transition into adulthood and become more independent, the health care team needs to help them maintain effective diabetes self-management skills.

Diabetes in women of childbearing age

Major congenital malformations remain the leading cause of mortality and serious morbidity in infants of mothers with pre-existing type 1 and type 2 diabetes. The risk of malformations increases continuously with increasing maternal glycemia during the first six to eight weeks of gestation. To minimize the occurrence of these devastating malformations, all women with diabetes who have childbearing potential should be counseled about:

- The risk of malformations associated with unplanned pregnancies and poor diabetes control and
- Use of effective contraception at all times, unless their diabetes is well managed and they are actively trying to conceive [1]

Because of the risk of gestational diabetes to the mother and neonate, screening, diagnosis, and effective treatment is necessary. Gestational diabetes increases infant macrosomia and adverse perinatal outcomes including caesarean section, spontaneous preterm delivery, shoulder dystocia or birth injury, neonatal hypoglycemia, and need for intensive neonatal care. [46] Women with a history of gestational diabetes are at lifelong increased risk for diabetes. The child of a diabetes pregnancy is at increased risk for obesity and diabetes later in life. See Table 5 for screening recommendations for women with history of gestational diabetes.

Women with diabetes or history of gestational diabetes who are planning pregnancy need to be seen frequently by a skilled multidisciplinary team experienced in the management of diabetes, before and during pregnancy. The management team will need to maintain stable blood glucose values close to normal, as well as identify and manage any existing long-term diabetic complications.

Diabetes in older adults

At least 20 percent of people over the age of 65 have diabetes. Older people with diabetes have higher rates of premature death, functional disability, and coexisting illnesses such as hypertension, coronary heart disease, and stroke than those without diabetes. Older adults with diabetes are also at greater risk than other older adults for several common geriatric syndromes, such as polypharmacy, depression, cognitive impairment, urinary incontinence, injurious falls, and persistent pain. While glycemic control has not been proven to reduce CVD in older

patients, there is strong evidence for lipid and blood pressure management.

Management goals therefore must be individualized. Older adults who are free of cardiovascular disease, active, cognitively intact, and willing to participate in self-management should be encouraged to do so and should be treated using the same goals for younger adults with diabetes. Older adults can be treated with the same medications as younger people, but special care is required in prescribing and monitoring therapy. Medications should be started at the lowest dose and titrated up gradually until targets are reached or side effects develop.

The family needs education to help older family members achieve their diabetes management goals and access useful resources.

Diabetes in high-risk racial groups

A number of racial and ethnic populations are disproportionately affected by diabetes. Compared to non-Hispanic white adults, African Americans, Hispanic/Latino Americans, and Asian Americans and Pacific Islanders are almost two times more likely to have diabetes. American Indians and Alaska Natives are more than two times as likely to have diabetes.

To provide optimal diabetes care, the health care team needs to learn how patients view and treat diabetes within their respective cultures. A practical approach to avoid stereotyping involves treating each patient encounter as unique and asking questions that elicit the patient's perspective on diagnosis and management such as "What is hardest for you about having diabetes?" or "Do you have any religious or family customs that affect how you care for your health?" This patient-centered approach enables collaboration and negotiation between the patient and health care team to develop and implement an effective diabetes management plan that addresses individual needs and customs. It is important that appropriate and culturally sensitive diabetes education materials are provided to all patients.

It is important to use appropriate A1C assay in people with hemoglobinopathy. See Sickle Cell Trait and Other Hemoglobinopathies and Diabetes: Important Information for Physician.
www.diabetes.niddk.nih.gov/dm/pubs/hemovari-A1C/.

Note. The Office of Minority Health provides resources to protect the health of racial and ethnic minority populations and eliminate health disparities: *www.omhrc.gov.*

Provide Regular Assessments to Monitor Treatment Effectiveness and to Detect Diabetes Complications

People with diabetes should have regular exams to monitor the effects of treatment, assess disease progression, and help find and treat diabetes complications. Assessment should be made on a regular basis using current, reliable methods. All diabetes complications have effective treatments.

Regular monitoring of diabetes management enables the diabetes team to assess achievement of treatment goals and to adjust therapy as necessary. Regular checking for long-term complications can help detect problems at a time when they can be treated and managed successfully. The physical examination, laboratory tests, and other assessments that the team conducts to monitor management and to identify complications early should be performed during routine diabetes visits, and at quarterly and annual visits.

At each diabetes visit:

- Measure weight, blood pressure, and calculate BMI.
- Inspect feet for lesions or abnormalities if one or more high-risk foot conditions are present.
- Review self-monitoring glucose record.
- Review/adjust medications to control glucose, lipids, blood pressure. Include regular use of low dose aspirin (if there are not contraindications) for cardiovascular disease prevention, as appropriate.
- Review self-management skills, progress toward behavior change goals, dietary needs, and physical activity as indicated.
- Assess for coping, depression, or other mood disorder.
- Counsel on smoking cessation and alcohol use.
- Review interventions for weight loss.

Quarterly:

- Obtain A1C in patients whose therapy has changed or who are not meeting glycemic goals (twice a year if at goal with stable glycemia).

Annually:

- Obtain fasting lipid profile (every two years if patient has low-risk lipid values).
- Obtain serum creatinine to estimate glomerular filtration rate and stage the level of chronic kidney disease.
- Perform urine test for albumin-to-creatinine ratio in patients with type 1 diabetes more than five years and in all patients with type 2 diabetes.
- Refer for dilated eye exam by an ophthalmologist or optometrist to detect retinal and other eye complications. If normal and the patient is not at high risk, the eye care specialist may advise an exam every two to three years.
- Perform comprehensive foot exam to check circulation, sensation, lesions, or changes in shape, and identify high-risk feet.
- Refer for dental/oral exam at least once a year to prevent periodontal disease, mouth infections, and loss of teeth.
- Administer influenza vaccination.
- Review need for other preventive care or treatment.

Lifetime:

- Administer pneumococcal vaccination (repeat if over 64 or immunocompromised and last vaccination was more than 5 years ago).

Resources

All NDEP materials are available free of charge.
To order, visit www.YourDiabetesInfo.org or call
1-888-693-NDEP (6337). Materials may be downloaded,
reproduced, and distributed without copyright restrictions.
Organization logos and contact information may be added
to NDEP materials for personal printing and distribution
needs.

Campaigns

Based on these guiding principles for diabetes care,
NDEP promotes early and intensive diabetes management
and prevention through widespread education campaigns
and community outreach programs. The *Control Your
Diabetes. For Life.* campaign promotes optimal comprehensive diabetes management. The *Small Steps. Big
Rewards. Prevent type 2 Diabetes.* campaign addresses
the need to prevent type 2 diabetes.

Materials for health care professionals — primary
care providers, diabetes educators, dietitians, nurses, pharmacists, and specialists, among many others, as well as
school personnel — all of whom need to be engaged in
caring for people with or at risk for diabetes. Materials
include:

Presentation slides

❏ *Diabetes: The Science of Control; Diabetes: The
Science of Prevention*
Slides sets present current information about diabetes
prevalence and incidence in the United States, and
diabetes management and prevention.

Quick reference materials

❏ *Diabetes Numbers At-a-Glance Reference Card*
A pocket guide provides a list of current recommendations to diagnose and manage pre-diabetes and
diabetes.

Diabetes management resources

❏ *Feet Can Last a Lifetime Kit*
A comprehensive foot care guide provides tools and
techniques to implement effective clinical procedures
and preventive foot care for people with diabetes.

❏ *Helping the Student with Diabetes Succeed.
A Guide for School Personnel*
A school guide helps the student, school personnel,
parents, and the health care team work together to
provide optimal diabetes management in the school
setting.

❏ *Si Tiene Diabetes, Cuide Su Corazón (If You
Have Diabetes, Take Care of Your Heart)*
A bilingual presentation flipchart (in Spanish and
English) helps educate Hispanic/Latino Americans
about the link between diabetes and heart disease.

❏ *Team Care: Comprehensive Lifetime
Management for Diabetes*
A team care booklet helps implement multidisciplinary team care for people with diabetes in various
settings.

❏ *Working Together to Manage Diabetes: Diabetes
Medications Supplement*
A detailed reference booklet profiles medications
used to manage blood glucose, blood pressure, and
cholesterol.

❏ *Working Together to Manage Diabetes: A Guide
for Pharmacists, Podiatrists, Optometrists, and
Dental Professionals*
An interdisciplinary primer focuses on diabetes-
related conditions affecting the foot, eye, and mouth,
as well as the issues related to medication management.

Diabetes prevention resources

❏ *Small Steps. Big Rewards. Your GAME PLAN
to Prevent Type 2 Diabetes: Health Care Provider
Toolkit*
A toolkit contains a decision pathway to diagnose and
treat pre-diabetes, proven strategies to counsel and
motivate patients, an office poster, and copier-ready
patient education materials.

❏ *The Road to Health Toolkit*
A multi-component primary prevention toolkit
provides several tools to promote type 2 diabetes
prevention through lifestyle change education that
focuses on healthy eating and increased physical
activity. CD/DVDs and training guide and video
included.

Materials for health care professionals to provide to their patients — NDEP work group members and partners, as well as focus group findings, help NDEP develop appropriate, culturally sensitive patient education materials and community partnership guides. Many of these materials help people learn about the seriousness of diabetes, ways to prevent and manage diabetes, and the resulting benefits.

Materials have been adapted for 21 different audiences: African American, American Indian and Alaska Native, 15 Asian and Pacific Islander audiences (in their languages), children and adolescents, older adults, Spanish speaking populations, and women with a history of gestational diabetes.

❑ *4 Steps to Control Your Diabetes for Life*, an easy to read booklet, is available in English and Spanish. It condenses these guiding principles and helps people with diabetes make informed decisions about their diabetes care.

❑ The *Small Steps. Big Rewards. Your GAME PLAN to Prevent Type 2 Diabetes* is an easy-to-read toolkit in English and — coming soon in Spanish — that helps people at risk take steps to prevent diabetes. Many tip sheets, tailored for multicultural audiences, older adults, and women with a history of gestational diabetes, help motivate patients to lose weight and increase their physical activity — small steps needed to achieve the big reward of preventing type 2 diabetes.

For more information about NDEP's partners, messages, campaigns, and materials, visit www.YourDiabetesInfo. org.

Additional websites

www.BetterDiabetesCare.nih.gov — provides tools and resources to help health care professionals identify and implement important changes in the delivery of diabetes care to improve patient outcomes.

www.DiabetesAtWork.org — provides tools and resources to help businesses and managed care organizations reduce diabetes risk factors in employees, assess the impact of diabetes in the workplace, and help employees manage diabetes and lower heart disease risk.

For more information on diabetes and related topics, visit the National Institute of Diabetes and Digestive and Kidney Diseases at www.niddk.nih.gov.

References

1. American Diabetes Association: Standards of medical care in diabetes—2009. Diabetes Care 2009; 32(Suppl 1): S13-61.

2. Centers for Disease Control and Prevention: National diabetes fact sheet: general information and national estimates on diabetes in the United States, 2007. 2008.

3. National Heart Lung and Blood Institute: Practical guide to the identification, evaluation and treatment of overweight and obesity in adults. Bethesda, MD: National Institutes of Health, 2000.

4. American Association of Clinical Endocrinologists medical guidelines for clinical practice for the management of diabetes mellitus. Endocr Pract 2007; 13(Suppl 1): 1-68.

5. United States Preventive Services Task Force: Guide to Clinical Preventive Services. 2nd ed. Alexandria, VA: Office of Disease Prevention and Health Promotion, 1996.

6. Metzger BE, Buchanan TA, Coustan DR, et al.: Summary and Recommendations of the Fifth International Workshop-Conference on Gestational Diabetes Mellitus. Diabetes Care 2007; 30(S2): S251-S260.

7. Knowler WC, Barrett-Connor E, Fowler SE, et al.: Reduction in the incidence of type 2 diabetes with lifestyle intervention or metformin. N Engl J Med 2002; 346(6): 393-403.

8. Pettitt DJ, Knowler WC: Long-term effects of the intrauterine environment, birth weight, and breast-feeding in Pima Indians. Diabetes Care 1998; 21(Suppl 2): B138-41.

9. Nathan DM, Davidson MB, DeFronzo RA, et al.: Impaired fasting glucose and impaired glucose tolerance: implications for care. Diabetes Care 2007; 30(3): 753-9.

10. National Heart Lung and Blood Institute/National Institute for Diabetes and Digestive and Kidney Diseases: Clinical guidelines on the identification, evaluation, and treatment of overweight and obesity in adults: the evidence report. Bethesda, MD: National Institutes of Health, 1998.

11. Inge TH, Krebs NF, Garcia VF, et al.: Bariatric surgery for severely overweight adolescents: concerns and recommendations. Pediatrics 2004; 114(1): 217-23.

12. Snow V, Barry P, Fitterman N, Qaseem A, Weiss K: Pharmacologic and surgical management of obesity in primary care: a clinical practice guideline from the American College of Physicians. Ann Intern Med 2005; 142(7): 525-31.

13. Funnell MM, Brown TL, Childs BP, et al.: National standards for diabetes self-management education. Diabetes Care 2007; 30(6): 1630-7.

14. Fisher EB, Brownson CA, O'Toole ML, et al.: The Robert Wood Johnson Foundation Diabetes Initiative: demonstration projects emphasizing self-management. Diabetes Educ 2007; 33(1): 83-4, 86-8, 91-2, passim.

15. Diabetes Control and Complications Trial Research Group: The effect of intensive treatment of diabetes on the development and progression of long-term complications in insulin-dependent diabetes mellitus. N Eng J Med 1993; 329(14): 977-86.

16. Nathan DM, Cleary PA, Backlund JY, et al.: Intensive diabetes treatment and cardiovascular disease in patients with type 1 diabetes. N Engl J Med 2005; 353(25): 2643-53.

17. Holman RR, Paul SK, Bethel MA, Matthews DR, Neil HA: 10-Year Follow-up of Intensive Glucose Control in Type 2 Diabetes. N Engl J Med 2008; 359(15): 1577-89.

18. Gerstein HC, Miller ME, Byington RP, et al.: Effects of intensive glucose lowering in type 2 diabetes. N Engl J Med 2008; 358(24): 2545-59.

19. Patel A, MacMahon S, Chalmers J, et al.: Intensive blood glucose control and vascular outcomes in patients with type 2 diabetes. N Engl J Med 2008; 358(24): 2560-72.

20. Duckworth W, Abraira C, Moritz T, et al.: Glucose control and vascular complications in veterans with type 2 diabetes. N Engl J Med 2009; 360(2): 129-39.

21. UK Prospective Diabetes Study (UKPDS) Group: Tight blood pressure control and risk of macrovascular and microvascular complications in type 2 diabetes: UKPDS 38. UK Prospective Diabetes Study Group. BMJ 1998; 317(7160): 703-13.

22. Holman RR, Paul SK, Bethel MA, Neil HA, Matthews DR: Long-Term Follow-up after Tight Control of Blood Pressure in Type 2 Diabetes. N Engl J Med 2008.

23. Hansson L, Zanchetti A, Carruthers SG, et al.: Effects of intensive blood-pressure lowering and low-dose aspirin in patients with hypertension: principal results of the Hypertension Optimal Treatment (HOT) randomised trial. HOT Study Group. Lancet 1998; 351(9118): 1755-62.

24. Kostis JB, Wilson AC, Freudenberger RS, Cosgrove NM, Pressel SL, Davis BR: Long-term effect of diuretic-based therapy on fatal outcomes in subjects with isolated systolic hypertension with and without diabetes. Am J Cardiol 2005; 95(1): 29-35.

25. Heart Outcomes Prevention Evaluation Study Investigators: Effects of ramipril on cardiovascular and microvascular outcomes in people with diabetes mellitus: results of the HOPE study and the MICRO-HOPE substudy. Lancet 2000; 355: 253-9.

26. Niskanen L, Hedner T, Hansson L, Lanke J, Niklason A: Reduced cardiovascular morbidity and mortality in hypertensive diabetic patients on first-line therapy with an ACE inhibitor compared with a diuretic/beta-blocker-based treatment regimen: a subanalysis of the Captopril Prevention Project. Diabetes Care 2001; 24(12): 2091-6.

27. Nielsen FS, Rossing P, Gall MA, Skott P, Smidt UM, Parving HH: Impact of lisinopril and atenolol on kidney function in hypertensive NIDDM subjects with diabetic nephropathy. Diabetes 1994; 43(9): 1108-13.

28. Patel A, MacMahon S, Chalmers J, et al.: Effects of a fixed combination of perindopril and indapamide on macrovascular and microvascular outcomes in patients with type 2 diabetes mellitus (the ADVANCE trial): a randomised controlled trial. Lancet 2007; 370(9590): 829-40.

29. American Diabetes Association: Management of dyslipidemia in adults with diabetes. Diabetes Care 2000; 23(Suppl.1): S57-S60.

30. Goldberg RB, Mellies MJ, Sacks FM, et al.: Cardiovascular events and their reduction with pravastatin in diabetic and glucose-intolerant myocardial infarction survivors with average cholesterol levels: subgroup analyses in the cholesterol and recurrent events (CARE) trial. The Care Investigators. Circulation 1998; 98(23): 2513-9.

31. Sacks FM, Pfeffer MA, Moye LA, et al.: The effect of pravastatin on coronary events after myocardial infarction in patients with average cholesterol levels. Cholesterol and Recurrent Events Trial investigators. N Engl J Med 1996; 335(14): 1001-9.

32. Haffner SM, Alexander CM, Cook TJ, et al.: Reduced coronary events in simvastatin-treated patients with coronary heart disease and diabetes or impaired fasting glucose levels: subgroup analyses in the Scandinavian Simvastatin Survival Study. Arch Intern Med 1999; 159(22): 2661-7.

33. Colhoun HM, Betteridge DJ, Durrington PN, et al.: Primary prevention of cardiovascular disease with atorvastatin in type 2 diabetes in the Collaborative Atorvastatin Diabetes Study (CARDS): multicentre randomised placebo-controlled trial. Lancet 2004; 364(9435): 685-96.

34. Gaede P, Vedel P, Larsen N, Jensen GV, Parving HH, Pedersen O: Multifactorial intervention and cardiovascular disease in patients with type 2 diabetes. N Engl J Med 2003; 348(5): 383-93.

35. Gaede P, Lund-Andersen H, Parving HH, Pedersen O: Effect of a multifactorial intervention on mortality in type 2 diabetes. N Engl J Med 2008; 358(6): 580-91.

36. Pi-Sunyer X, Blackburn G, Brancati FL, et al.: Reduction in weight and cardiovascular disease risk factors in individuals with type 2 diabetes: one-year results of the look AHEAD trial. Diabetes Care 2007; 30(6): 1374-83.

37. Skyler JS, Bergenstal R, Bonow RO, et al.: Intensive glycemic control and the prevention of cardiovascular events: implications of the ACCORD, ADVANCE, and VA diabetes trials: a position statement of the American Diabetes Association and a scientific statement of the American College of Cardiology Foundation and the American Heart Association. Diabetes Care 2009; 32(1): 187-92.

38. A comprehensive assessment of North American and United Kingdom glycemic control guidelines. Ann Intern Med 2007; 147(6): 417-22 &152.

39. Nathan DM, Buse JB, Davidson MB, et al.: Management of hyperglycemia in type 2 diabetes: a consensus algorithm for the initiation and adjustment of therapy: a consensus statement from the American Diabetes Association and the European Association for the Study of Diabetes. Diabetes Care 2008; 31(12): 1-11.

40. Nathan DM, Kuenen J, Borg R, et al.: Translating the A1C assay into estimated average glucose values. Diabetes Care 2008; 31(8): 1473-1478.

41. Bolen S, Feldman L, Vassy J, et al.: Systematic review: comparative effectiveness and safety of oral medications for type 2 diabetes mellitus. Ann Intern Med 2007; 147(6): 386-99.

42. Bantle JP, Wylie-Rosett J, Albright AL, et al.: Nutrition recommendations and interventions for diabetes: a position statement of the American Diabetes Association. Diabetes Care 2008; 31(Suppl 1): S61-78.

43. American Diabetes Association: Clinical Practice Recommendations -Standards of Medical Care in Diabetes. Diabetes Care 2007; 30(Suppl. 1): S4-S41.

44. Sigal RJ, Kenny GP, Wasserman DH, Castaneda-Sceppa C, White RD: Physical activity/exercise and type 2 diabetes: a consensus statement from the American Diabetes Association. Diabetes Care 2006; 29(6): 1433-8.

45. Rodriguez BL, Fujimoto WY, Mayer-Davis EJ, et al.: Prevalence of cardiovascular disease risk factors in U.S. children and adolescents with diabetes: the SEARCH for diabetes in youth study. Diabetes Care 2006; 29(8): 1891-6.

46. Metzger BE, Lowe LP, Dyer AR, et al.: Hyperglycemia and adverse pregnancy outcomes. N Engl J Med 2008; 358(19): 1991-2002.

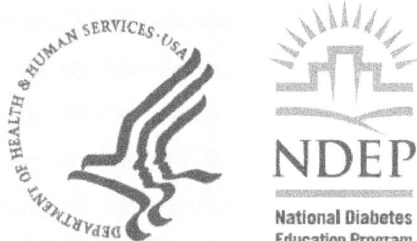

The U.S. Department of Health and Human Services' National Diabetes Education Program is jointly sponsored by the National Institutes of Heath and the Centers for Disease Control and Prevention with the support of more than 200 partner organizations.

www.YourDiabetesInfo.org   1-888-693-NDEP (6337)   TTY: 1-866-569-1162

NIH Publication No. 09-4343   NDEP-16   Revised April 2009